The Ultimate Guide To Overcome Alcohol Addiction For Life

The Most Effective, Permanent Solution To Finally Cure Alcoholism

John K.

Table of Contents

Introduction

I want to thank you and congratulate you for purchasing the book, *"The Ultimate Guide to Overcome Alcohol Addiction for Life: The Most Effective, Permanent Solution to Finally Cure Alcoholism"*.

This book contains proven steps and strategies on how to overcome alcohol addiction, which is difficult if not almost impossible to defeat. But too much of alcohol—or of anything—is not good for the body, the soul, and the mind. There has to be a way to be able to defeat alcoholism and be free from this addiction.

This book centers on the secrets of how to overcome alcohol abuse and addiction. Many people have tried to stop their alcohol intake, especially those who are becoming addicted to it. However, changing habits are as difficult as changing the world. The secret lies on the ability to see things differently, with the belief that they are indeed capable of fulfilling their desires, no matter how difficult.

Thanks again for purchasing this book, I hope you enjoy it!

Chapter 1: What is alcohol addiction?

"Alcohol addiction"—or what is referred to as alcoholism—indicates a dependency on the intake of alcohol that affects the physical and psychological systems of the human body. Because alcohol can be an addictive substance, people may find themselves wanting more and more of it, and they also tend to lose their self-control while being under the power of the liquor. Alcohol addiction is something that has to be overcome, or else they may lose their capacity to think straight and be able to harness their growth.

It is important to note that "alcohol addiction" is different from "alcohol abuse". The former refers to the tendency to want more and more, together with the tendency to lose one's self-control and the ability to disallow the intake of alcohol. "Alcohol abuse", on the other hand, refers to the act of drinking more than what is needed regardless of the results. Thus, those who tend to abuse their intake of alcohol may not be addicted to it and may only drink alcohol about once a week. To experience alcohol abuse does not necessarily mean they are experiencing alcohol addiction as well, as they are very different from one another. However, there is the heavy tendency that those who abuse alcohol would later on become dependent on it, resulting to alcohol addiction in the latter period.

It is said that alcoholism is the result of many interconnected factors that had taken place in the past and the present of the person affected. It includes important factors, such as genetics, emotional health, social environment, and the manner in which the person was raised or trained. Findings suggest that there is greater tendency for people to become alcohol addicted when they are raised witnessing the intake of alcohol from other people, especially those who were close to the person. This includes the family, relatives, and close friends, not to mention their associates and those whom the person idolizes during their early years or when they were still young. This is because people have the tendency to follow their instincts, and instincts suggest that what people see in their surroundings they tend to follow and apply in real life. Thus, people who have a family history of alcoholism are usually the ones who develop drinking problems.

Some races are likewise more at risk of experiencing alcohol addiction, such as the American Indians and the Native Alaskans. It also includes those who have mental health problems, such as anxiety, depression, as well as bipolar disorder. Because alcohol can be used for self-medication, people with mental health problems are at risk of experiencing alcohol addiction, as they may tend to use alcohol to bring instant relief from anxiety, grief, tension, anger, and depression.

There are a number of signs that are prevalent whenever a person is experiencing drinking problems or alcohol addiction. Most people who are experiencing alcohol addiction usually feel guilty or ashamed about their habits of drinking, and they tend to defend themselves too much, as if people are harassing them for their habits of drinking too much alcohol. They also tend to lie to people, saying that they are not engaged in alcoholism and are never addicted to alcohol... or any type of substance for that matter. They tend to hide their drinking habits and they make sure that nobody would witness them lest they would be convicted of being a loser—one who cannot control his or her intake, one who is weak and has no capacity to reject alcohol.

Another sign that a person is having drinking problems is the fact that close friends and family members are starting to get worried about the person drinking too much alcohol. Many people are starting to notice that the amount of alcohol being drunk is a little too way over the boundary. Meanwhile, another sign of a person experiencing alcohol addiction is that, there is a certain comfort or relief that is felt when drinking alcohol for a certain period. The person feels much better, as if he/she is more relaxed and more at rest whenever he/she drinks alcohol. Thus, he/she does it more often, since there is a feeling of relief whenever the person drinks alcohol. The person would just find himself or herself drinking more than what he/she intends to. With the person drinking more than what is intended, there is the tendency to forget what took place during the drinking session—a sign that the amount of alcohol intake was too much than what was considered normal to drink.

In a matter of time, people who start to abuse their intake of alcohol would normally find them experiencing problems, as a result of taking too much alcohol. That would be another sign that the person is having drinking problems. Drinking alcohol for social gatherings is considered acceptable. However, to drink more than what is intended would not be good for the person, as it may create problems in the family and the society, since too much alcohol intake can lead to rude and careless words and actions, which can directly affect other people. It can likewise affect the person's relationship with other people. It can affect the person's job and financial condition while, at the same time, affect his/her state of security and his/her state of wellbeing. When these things happen, it is time to do something to overcome alcohol addiction, as it may lead to mental, emotional, and psychological problems that can lead to destruction.

Chapter 2: Change the way you think

In any type of problem, the first step is to acknowledge what is presently happening, and to accept what the person has done and what is being done as of the moment. They have to admit that they have currently wronged the use of alcohol and have instead, abused the use of it, which led to alcohol abuse and addiction. People have to acknowledge and accept first what they have done in the past so that they would have the clarity of mind to see where they are currently standing and what has happened to them because of that thing that was done. There has to be the initiative to see where they currently are, and to have the conviction to be where they should be or to do what they should rightfully do. Without this initiative, there will be no desire to see the present, which would prevent them from seeing their future prospect, in connection to their abuse of alcohol intake. The first step therefore, is to create a purpose by means of rational thought, to understand that by abusing the intake of alcohol they have committed a mistake, which they should alter because it is not good and not healthy for them. As one expert in this subject have said, a person will eventually lead to nowhere if he or she is denial about it, minimizing it and belittling it like it is not one of the most important things that had to be refurbished in life.

Once a person has entered into rational thought, it is time to acknowledge a purpose. They should try to think why they should do it, why they should drink tons of alcohol for an unlimited time. What is the purpose or the objective for that act that they are doing? Is there something good that they would profit out of drinking too much alcohol over a period of time? Are there some benefits? What are they? They should try and meditate over the act of alcohol intake that they are presently experiencing, and see what the advantages the action brings to them as a person. This is the time for meditation, when the person begins to ask about the main purpose the action is being subjected to. They have to realize that they do not just drink because they are thirsty, but because of the effect of anxiety, depression, as well as pain. They are looking for something that would numb them from these negative emotions, and they have found the answer in a bottle of alcohol. Once they have acknowledged these things, it will be clear why they are doing it and what they really want to do, whether they want to continue doing it or maybe one day stop doing it. The purpose will become more evident, as they are able to understand more their reason for doing it.

After the person has acknowledged the purpose, it is then time to create a mission that is: to try and stop alcohol addiction once and for all. They have to choose to overcome alcohol addiction. No one will push them to stop alcohol addiction. It is up to them to choose whether they want to continue or if they want to stop it. They have to understand that what happens to them is everything that they have wanted to happen to them. No one else can tell them to do this or to engage in this; to stop this or to give this up. Even if all their relatives and friends are there to support them as they give up alcohol addiction, everything and everyone will be useless unless the person decides to stop it themselves, to do it themselves. If they do not choose to do it, then nobody can do it for them. Thus, they have to choose to overcome alcohol addiction. They have to see why they have to stop this abuse of alcohol intake, and what leads them to become, as a result of alcohol abuse and addiction. As it is said, the biggest leverage in the lives of people can be found in the hearts and in the minds. There is nobody who can eliminate these things from their lives but them and only them.

Meanwhile, it is important to think that, what people intend to become they will soon become. It is important to experience the *theory of expectancy*, wherein people develop the belief that, what they want to become, they will soon become. They have to believe that if they want to stop alcohol abuse and addiction, then time will come when they will finally see these things as events of the past. There will no longer be alcoholism in their lives but only the courage to take what is only necessary—just enough for the time being, enough for the body, enough for the mind. If people have certain expectancy with regards to their initiative, then that objective will become easier to handle, no matter how difficult it is for the time being. In time, they will get motivated to continue doing what they feel they should do, as they can visualize themselves in light, wherein they successfully get over their difficulties in life, especially when it comes to alcoholism. The first step therefore, is to tune in their thoughts and their minds, to make sure that they are concentrated on accomplishing their task, no matter how difficult it seemed.

Chapter 3: Change the way you live

After the person has changed the way he or she thinks, it is time to change the way he or she lives. This is the time when what they have thought of, they do it with conviction. They do not just create a mission or an objective but that they *do* something about the objective that they have created. Thus, at this point, it is time to create a plan, which the person does, to make sure that they would be able to fulfill their objective, which is to stop alcohol addiction and abuse. At this stage, they create strategies that would lead them to overcoming their alcohol addiction.

For instance, it would be good to create alternative coping skills, as they face this difficulty of trying to give up the habit of taking more alcohol than what is really necessary. These coping skills can be done by making sure that bad habits are being replaced by good ones. As it has been said, bad habits are not broken but are being replaced with new ones. Thus, these alternative skills may include the initiative of trying to recognize their rewards for trying to quit drinking. Rewards are really useful, especially when people face tasks that are quite difficult to achieve over a period of time.

They should think of what they will soon get once they have succeeded in lessening their intake of alcohol, once they develop the ability of being able to control their cravings. Experts have mentioned the necessity of having positive thoughts when trying to fulfill tasks. They said that these positive thoughts can calm the minds of people, and it can take away the anxiety and the worry of not knowing how to start or end the task. It can lift the spirit and give an inspiring message both to the mind and the spirit, that the pain may be removed in replacement of something that is more worthwhile to think of and to possess. As it is once said, one cannot just take something away without putting something in replacement of it. There has to be something to fill up the emptiness and the vacancy, for in this the coping mechanisms begins to work out, and the person will not be going back to where he or she has been before the dilemma began taking place.

Secondly, it is important to make lifestyle changes. These would start in the little things that the person does, such as cleaning their cupboards of all the alcoholic beverages that once were aligned in a variety. They can also try to prevent going to parties or drinking sessions, wherein they tend to drink alcohol with their friends and associates. They may also try not to go to the clubs, or even their friends' house, where they tend to drink alcohol without limit. Likewise, they may try to drink black coffee instead, whenever they feel like trying to drink another bottle of alcohol. Others would rather smoke some cigarettes, just to take away the cravings. All these may be little things, but they all mean a lot, especially when it comes to doing something that is really difficult to do or to achieve. Trying to overcome alcohol addiction is really difficult to achieve, which may be the reason why others would rather try and stop doing it with another friend or family member. Others do not do it alone. Instead, they find another person who is close to them, and they do their mission with this person and share with them their difficulties and what they have achieved so far. If another person is doing fine in his or her mission of trying to overcome alcohol addiction, the other one may become more motivated to give up drinking alcohol, since another person is doing the same task, meaning they are not alone in their ordeal. They have another person to express their difficulties with and what they have experienced so far, and that alone can give them the strength to overcome something that is difficult to give up, such as alcohol abuse and addiction.

Meanwhile, it would be best to use rewards once the person has succeeded in his or her mission over some period of time. If, for example, they have succeeded in trying to abstain from drinking alcohol, say for two months, then they should give themselves some rewards for being able to do that, such as giving themselves a treat or going to the movie and celebrating the day, since they have succeeded in their mission. They should acknowledge that they have indeed succeeded in their first stage, and the second stage would be to continue it for another two months, for example. By giving themselves some rewards, they finally acknowledge that they are indeed, making progress, and they have to motivate themselves a little bit more to make sure they continue with their mission for the upcoming months. However, they should never think of their mission as something to be done in too lengthy a time. Instead, they should think of their mission in stages or in smaller periods of time, such as every six months. They should never think of their mission as one that corresponds to eternity, and never think that there will be no other way of drinking alcohol or that never again would they be able to taste it. They should just do it one step at a time… and things will happen as planned.

Chapter 4: Change the way you drink

After the person has changed the way he or she lives, it is time to change the way he or she drinks. This is very important, since the act itself has to be changed if the person really wants to prevent the abuse of alcohol, especially since he or she cannot assure that never again would he or she be able to drink liquor in the future. They have to know or to learn the right way of drinking liquor, to make sure that they have control over themselves whenever they drink liquor. Time will come when they will finally sit in front of a bottle of alcohol and ask themselves how in the world they should carry themselves. If they still have not learned how to rightfully drink alcohol, then the old ways will come again, and the abuse and addiction will again enter into their system, creating again the old problems that once they thought were already a thing of the past.

It has been well accepted that something that is a part of a person's past cannot be erased totally in one sweep. Instead, that thing should be eradicated from his or her life one step at a time. If this is about alcohol addiction, and the person usually takes alcohol for, let's say, twice a week, then the first step is to take it for only once a week for one month. After taking it once a week for one month, it is high time to take it every 10 days three times a month. After taking it every 10 days for a month, then it is high time to take it only twice a month every two weeks. After taking it only twice a month, then it is high time they should take it for only once a month... and then decrease the intake again and again until they would experience alcohol intake for, let's say, every two or three months. In time, that person will realize that he/she has not been taking alcohol for half a year, since he/she did it step by step, without thinking too much of his/her mission. In all these, it is evident that when trying to overcome alcohol addiction, the method is not to erase it once and for all, but to lessen the intake little by little, until such time when the alcohol intake transpires for only once or twice a year. In other words, people should know how to drink the right way—not to totally prevent him/her from drinking, but to drink liquor in the right manner.

On the other hand, when trying to overcome alcohol abuse, then they should try lessening their intake of alcohol little by little. If, for example, the person normally drinks eight bottles of alcohol in one drinking session, then the first step would be to decrease the number of bottles to six bottles, for example. The second step would be to decrease it again to four bottles of alcohol. The third step would be to decrease it again to three bottles, until the time comes whey they only have to drink two bottles of alcohol in one drinking session. In the same way, the answer is not to totally eradicate the intake of alcohol, but to lessen the intake little by little, one step at a time. Think of it little by little to prevent being too overwhelmed by the mission of lessening the intake of alcohol.

Meanwhile, it is likewise important that a person trying to overcome alcohol abuse and addiction should be able to identify the danger zones of when and where they are most likely to drink alcohol. These danger zones they should prevent by doing other things or going to other places, instead of being around those danger zones on those most dangerous times of the day. Say, for example, the danger zone is at 7 pm after the day is over and work has already been settled, then it would be better to do breathing exercises during that time of the day—something that will keep them from feeling the effect of not taking in liquor during that time of the day. They can also try doing some yoga or some relaxation activities right within the room.

Meanwhile, if the danger zone is at the house of a friend that they tend to pass by when going home from work, then it is high time to use another road when going home from work. As the experts have said, getting over the moments of impulse two or three times will eventually lead to a zero impulse, until there is no need to take in anything. People do not have to be strong the whole day through. They only need to know their strengths and weaknesses, and the time and place when they are most likely to be pressured and prompted to take again some alcohol. They have to know their danger zones so that they will be ready to face them with the right tactics—something that is incompatible with the addiction, as something that is difficult to overcome, such as alcohol, should be fought over. This means that people should be ready to face them square by square, especially during the most difficult time of the day when they feel instigated to again go back to their ritual of drinking alcohol. Once or twice, they may need to give themselves some break, but this should only take place when there is really nothing

that can be done—nothing to stop the cravings
for a little taste of liquor.

Chapter 5: Get support from others

After changing the manner of thinking, drinking, and living, it is high time to engage with the others in the community to avail some support so that they can achieve their goal of trying to eradicate alcohol addiction from their lives. People can drive support not only from their families and friends but also their associates around their communities, including those whom they deal with in the social networking sites and other discussion groups found in the Internet. Meanwhile, because alcohol abuse and addiction are already becoming a crisis in the society, there are already a number of organizations and community support groups that treat and help people who are locked within the walls of alcoholism. They are usually helpful when it comes to reinforcing positive transformation to people, even those who had been overpowered by alcohol abuse and addiction. They inspire continued positive belief within the individual, while giving them the ability to overcome something as strenuous as that of an addiction. They are mostly helpful to people who are negatively addicted, and it would be great to spend some time with them, as they can very well understand what a person trying to overcome an addiction really feels like. They know all the difficulties and know the best strategies that can be used in facing those difficulties.

By being in contact with a support system, a person trying to overcome alcohol abuse and addiction will have other people assisting them. This is very important, since it is never easy trying to stop something that has already been made a habit. Unlike friends and family, these people are more straightforward and tolerant, and they will tell that person directly if they are just kidding themselves or if everything is just turning out to be useless. There is no softness or feeling of coyness that prevents them from telling directly the truth. Instead, they say what should be said directly to the person, especially if it is for the best of him or her that the truth should be told. More so, having a support system allows other people to be engaged in the mission of trying to lessen the intake of alcohol. They may be helpful when telling friends that they should not be indulged in drinking alcohol, even during parties or during treats. With a support system, people trying to overcome alcohol addiction will have greater ability to maneuver the actions of other people, which may influence the person's act of drinking alcohol. The community will then embrace his or her decision to eradicate alcohol from his or her life, to live a more healthy life by controlling the intake of liquor. They will also know when it is the right time for the person to seek treatment, or when it is time to check into a rehabilitative program. A support system allows the supervision of alcohol discontinuity in the most flexible, deliberate manner, which can largely affect the mission of trying to stop the intake of alcohol by tapping in the external extremities in the society.

There are a number of alcohol treatment centers that are made available around the society nowadays. These alcohol treatment centers are all designed in helping people overcome their alcohol addiction, especially when it starts to affect their lives or when problems are starting to unfold as a result of drinking alcohol. Usually, these treatment centers require people to stay for a number of hours in which people who are addicted are given short- or long-term treatment options. Included in these options is the process of *detoxification*, wherein the alcohol is being removed from the body to get rid of the physical dependency of the person to the specific substance liquor. It is this detoxification that should begin to change the habit of drinking liquor, unless they do not drink alcohol on a regular basis or, in other words, if the person is not addicted to alcohol substance.

However, it is always important that people wanting to overcome alcohol abuse and addiction should very well understand why an abuse problem should be eradicated. They should understand that what they are going through is something that should not take place, and that it is unwise and unhealthy to drink too much alcohol in too often a time. Once they understand this, they undergo an individual therapy and a group therapy, in which they are made to understand their purpose for drinking alcohol and what the effects are, or how it affects their lives as a whole. They are made more conscious of what they can do to overcome their abusive behavior, and whether they really want to give this up for a better future. During a treatment program, people who are alcohol addicted are assisted with constructive ideas and alternatives for them to control their cravings and become more responsible with their actions. In due time, they can live a more productive lifestyle, as other people have assisted them in their mission of trying to overcome alcohol addiction on a day-to-day basis.

Chapter 6: Live for the future

When people engaged in overcoming alcohol addiction have changed the way they think, live, and drink, and they have acquired the support of treatment centers in the society, the last stage is to direct the soul and the mind onto the future. This is very important, since by directing the soul and the mind onto the future, the prospect is being shifted onto the future—forward and not backward. This prevents the person from being overwhelmed with all the strategies that should be done at the present time to successfully complete the mission and overcome alcohol addiction. It prevents the person from focusing on the past as well, which would only remind him or her of how alcohol can be abused, as proven in the past deeds. A new prospect and vision would have to be created so that there will be wider understanding on what deeds are deemed better and acceptable, in light of the new prospect that was created. The person would have to live for the future, not the past, so that there will be hope and renewed strength, which become sources of potency and control with regards to the corresponding mission. In this last stage, the vision is centered on creating a light of hope, and this light is centered on the future panorama, since it is the future that usually gives strength to people, especially during difficulties.

People who want to overcome alcohol addiction and abuse should let their future selves take control. They should allow a new self to be created within them, that by creating a new vision and a new mission, they become "new" and "fresh"—alive, with the spirit to do what is being intended, in spite of the difficulties. This creates a new self, wherein a new goal can be made, while pushing oneself to achieve these things, such as overcoming alcohol abuse and addiction. They just have to remember that there were times when they have proven themselves to be capable of fulfilling a new goal and a new mission. They have only set their minds to it, and they were able to achieve it, no matter how difficult and impossible it may have seemed. Now that the vision is centered on the future, there would be more chances of proving that, things that seemed impossible can be reached and fulfilled. Just believe in the capacity of the self. Be confident… and what seemed to be out of reach will eventually take place sooner or later. The answer only lies on the capacity of the self to believe, since it is by believing that the self is motivated to achieve what seemed desperately unattainable. Still, there is no way to believe and be motivated if the prospect is directed on the failures of the past. People have to center their vision on the future, for them to achieve growth and accomplishment. Then again, direct the eye not too far into the future, for it may overwhelm the person and lead him or her into a state of shock and desperation. Believe that it can be achieved… and soon it will be.

Conclusion

Thank you again for purchasing this book!

I hope this book was able to help you to overcome alcohol addiction for life. There are about 700,000 people who are being treated everyday due to problems in alcoholism. All of them wanted to be free from alcohol abuse and addiction; however, not all of them have achieved what they have wanted so far. The secret lies on the person's mind and soul, to create a "future self" that takes full control of oneself, one who can alter and redirect the manner of thinking, drinking, and living. In this future identity, things such as alcohol will be in their hands, and managing alcohol intake will be as simple as counting the trees.

The next step is to practicing what you have learned.

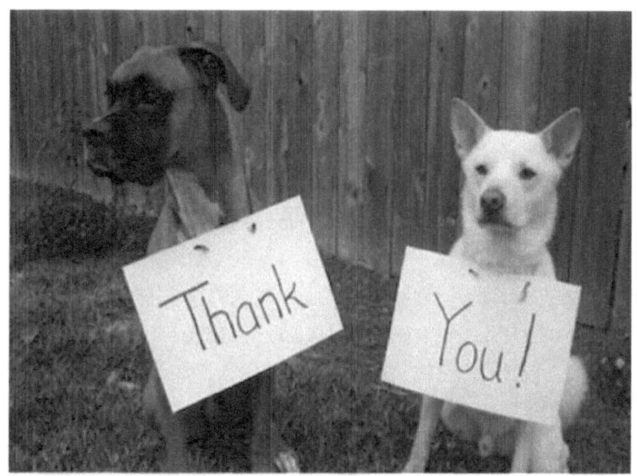

Finally, if you enjoyed this book, then I'd like to ask you for a favor, would you be kind enough to leave a review for this book on Amazon? It'd be greatly appreciated!

Thank you and good luck!

Check Out My Other Books

Below you'll find some of my other popular books that are popular on Amazon and Kindle as well. Simply click on the links below to check them out. Alternatively, you can visit my author page on Amazon to see other work done by me. If the links do not work, for whatever reason, you can simply search for these titles on the Amazon website to find them.

1) The Ultimate Guide To Become An Early Riser For Life - How To Awake Early And Be Productive Forever

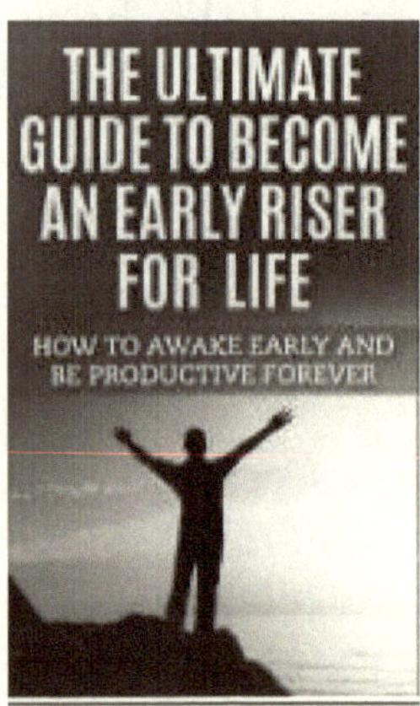

go to: http://amzn.to/1MRDEMr

2) The Ultimate Guide To Become An Alpha Male - How To Attract Women, Win In Life And Be Confident

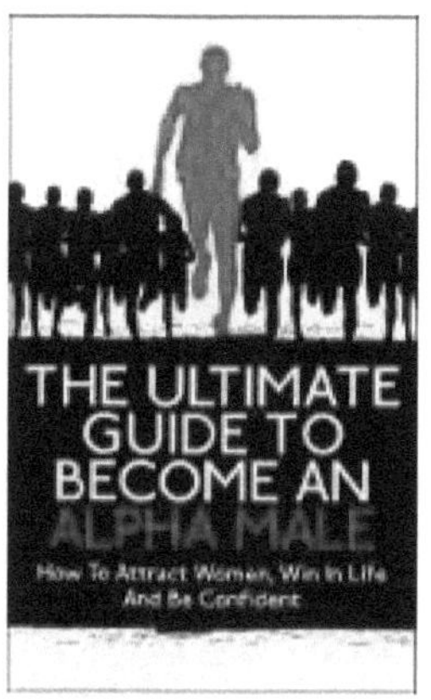

go to: http://amzn.to/20G8bBo

3) The Ultimate Guide To Honeymoon - How To Make Your Honeymoon Last Forever

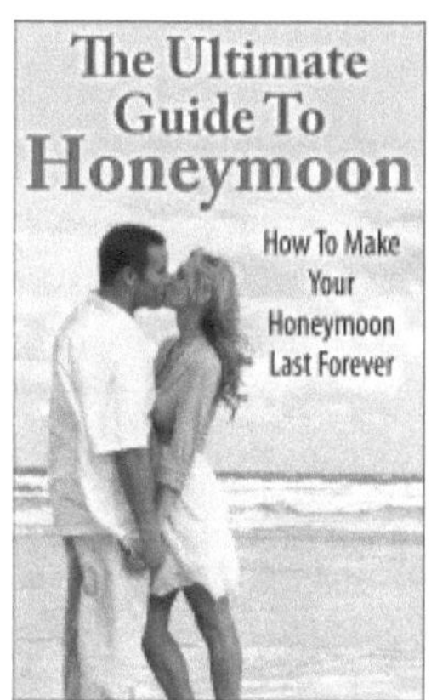

go to: http://amzn.to/1L7O6I9

4) The Drug Addiction Cure - The Most Effective, Permanent Solution to Finally Overcome Drug Addiction for Life

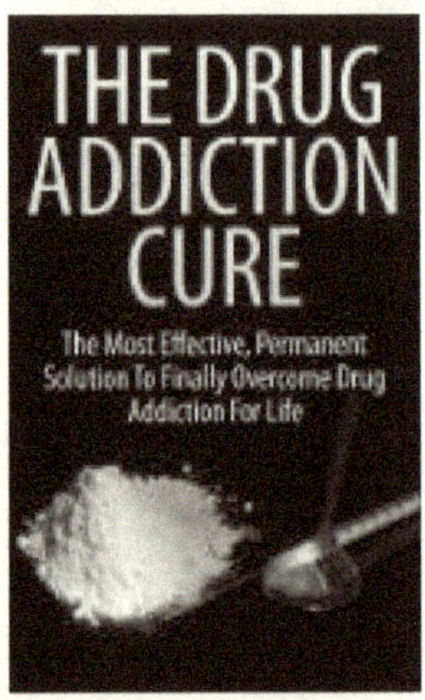

go to: http://amzn.to/1kkb9uc

5) How to Stop Snoring for Life - The Most Effective Cures and Remedies for Snoring

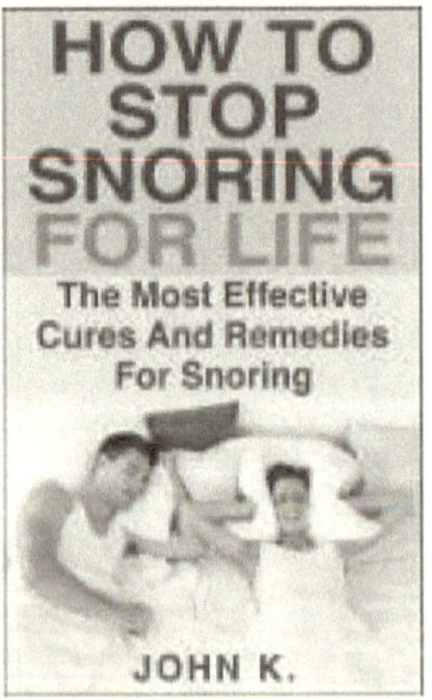

go to: http://amzn.to/1NE9uLn